Your Health

Originally Published in 1934 by Joseph H. Pilates

Prof. Pilates' Health Studios

Where flat feet, curvature of the spine, protruding stomach, stooped-shoulders, hollow chest, hollow back, bow legs, and knocked-kneed conditions are cured through corrective exercises.

Edited, Reformatted and Reprinted
in a New and Easy-to-Read Edition
by Presentation Dynamics
949-666-5030
ISBN13: 978-0-9614937-8-3

Updated with a new introduction by
Judd Robbins and Lin Van Heuit-Robbins
Copyright © 1998-2015 Presentation Dynamics Inc.
First Published in 1934 by Joseph H. Pilates

FOREWORD

All new ideas are revolutionary and when the theory responsible for them is proved, through practical application, it requires only time for them to develop and to flourish. Such revolutionary ideas simply cannot be ignored. They cannot be kept in the background.

Time and progress are synonymous terms-nothing can stop either.

Truth will prevail and that is why I know that my teachings will reach the masses and finally be adopted as universal.

INTRODUCTION

PERFECT Balance of Body and Mind, is that quality in civilized man, which not only gives him superiority over the savage and animal kingdom, but furnishes him with all the physical and mental powers that are indispensable for attaining the goal of Mankind -HEALTH and HAPPINESS.

The purpose of this booklet is to transmit in a simple form, the causes of present day ill-health and immoral conditions, and the resultant effects which prevent the average human being from attaining this physical perfection - man's inherited birthright.

The author in this booklet tries to teach the reader in simple words the way to correct our present deplorable system of physical and moral education, and to enable each, through a proper understanding of his body, to become fit for the daily tasks ahead of him.

JOSEPH HUBERTUS PILATES

2

INTRODUCTION
by Judd Robbins and Lin Van Heuit-Robbins

Joseph Pilates preached the benefits of a perfect balance of body and mind. He also followed his own teachings. He coupled his own gymnastics and martial arts background with a keen analytical approach to body mechanics, posture, and correct breathing. All of these background fundamentals appealed to us intellectually. When we began to experience his recommendations for exercises, postural modifications, and breathing mechanisms, we truly began to feel like converts.

Our own background in fitness and athletics began years ago with competitive high school and college athletics. Lin was a gymnast and Judd was a tennis and squash player. After college, Lin went on to design and teach a variety of programs in aerobics, stretching and flexibility, and weight training. She studied advanced methodologies in exercise physiology while obtaining a Masters Degree at the University of California at Berkeley, and also holds certifications in group fitness training and personal training from the American Council on Exercise (ACE). She has been for many years a reviewer for the ACE correspondence accreditation committee.

Judd combined a degree in physics with advanced degrees from the University of Michigan and the University of California at Berkeley to develop his own very analytical approach to exercise. He was a racquetball pro in the late '70s and has since earned a 3rd degree black belt in jujitsu plus a group fitness certification from the American Council on Exercise. Both Lin and Judd are certified by the PhysicalMind Institute in New York City in the matwork originally developed by Joseph and Clara Pilates.

There are many excellent books in the field of health, exercise, and fitness. We've read and use the principles offered in many of them, from yoga to stretching to strength training. We strongly believe that Joseph Pilates created a truly effective combination of strengthening and stretching that can work well for virtually every body. With the right instruction and guidance, some or all of Pilates' recommendations can demonstrably improve anybody's health and fitness levels.

TABLE OF CONTENTS

DEDICATION

TO:
The Next Generation of Physicians
and
The Association of Medico-Physical Research

by Joseph Hubertus Pilates

I take this means to thank my dear friend, Nat Fleischer, a leading American authority of sports and physical education, for his kind help and suggestions. He has given me added impetus to carry on my work for the betterment of mankind in the construction of corrective apparatus for proper body development. Also my sincere thanks to William J. Miller.

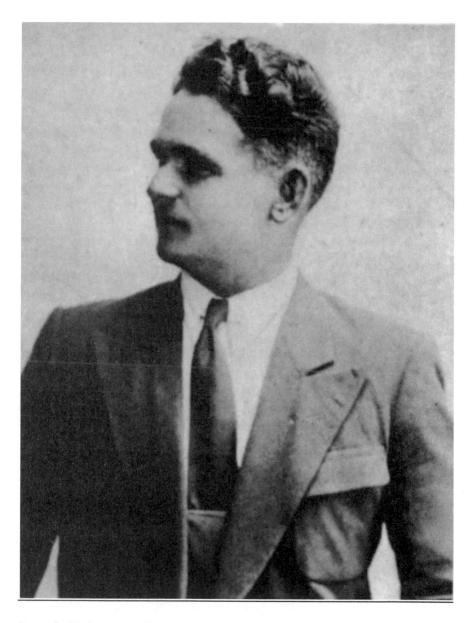

Joseph Hubertus Pilates: *This photograph was taken on his 54th birthday. He has devoted over thirty years to the scientific study, experimentation and research of disturbing troubles which upset Balance of Body and Mind*

5

Chapter 1: A Grave Situation

DAILY, from sunrise to sunset, the radio, newspapers and magazines broadcast to the world how to maintain health, how to regain health - what to eat, what to drink, and even about what to think.

The conflicting information, expressive of the different opinions of these various health authorities, has proved to be nothing less than "confusion worse confounded" to the millions of radio listeners, readers of newspapers and magazines, who are so unfortunate as to hear or read the diametrically opposed viewpoints of our so-called guardians of our health, since it is rather the exception than the rule, that these instructions are in agreement in their ideas and methods.

To one who has devoted the major portion of his life to the scientific study of the body and practical application of nature's laws of life as pertaining to the natural development of coordinated physical and mental (normal) health and the prevention, rather than the cure of disease, the misinformation he has so often listened to on the air or read, borders closely on the criminal. Why? Because the acceptance of the theories so advanced, not only results in the squandering of untold millions of dollars, but, what is more serious, results in actually shortening, instead of lengthening, the lives of uncounted millions who fall for this bunk.

How many hundreds of thousands die prematurely between the age range of 35 and 59 years, who should rightfully live from 20 to 40 years longer if they but understood and applied the natural laws of life to normal living? Daily we hear the cry for more hospitals, more sanitariums, more homes for the crippled, more lunatic asylums, more reformatories and more prisons!

Who is responsible for this sad, abominable condition?

Our so-called health authorities, whose remarks are accepted as law; our so-called scientists, whose statements are religiously accepted - they primarily are to blame because they fail in their mission to civilization!

In the practical universal world, ignorance of the little-understood and much less practiced natural laws of life as applied to normal living, lies the cause for the condition referred to, and I blame those in control of our health systems, for not correcting the evil.

Figures may or may not lie, but the statistics compiled by the United States Army, Navy and Marine Service in the World War, point the way to truth and warn us what health paths to choose and what by-paths to ill-health we should avoid. The record speaks for itself!

How much longer shall this grave situation continue?

Is not this vital question worthy of the closest attention? Should we not have a most vigorous' support of at least a select group of men adequately clothed with the proper official authority and imbued with the necessary inherent idealism to initiate a campaign for the purpose of devoting only a comparatively few hours to an impartial investigation of the merits of my claims herein set forth, even in the face of pessimists' predictions of their failure?

I have proved my case hundreds of times to my pupils and patients, but those who hate to see the old order cast aside, refuse to acknowledge the benefits of my system. That's why I've written this booklet, so that all who are interested, may read, digest and know what is wrong with the human race today and how its physical ills can be cured or prevented.

Through medicine? No! Through their own efforts, simple exercising, simple health rules that **CAN** be observed and **MUST** be observed.

The truth ultimately will burst through the clouds of ignorance and, once in the clear atmosphere, will shine forever in the blue sky of knowledge.

Truth will - must conquer.

Instead of pursuing a policy of passivism, aggressive action should and must be taken to bring to light my teachings of health, strength and happiness through proper corrective exercises. The living examples of former broken-down human beings — ill physically and mentally, but now perfect specimens of manhood and womanhood — speak volumes for my work. Investigate and see for yourself.

It is confidently asserted by me that the statements following, representing my personal views, can be demonstrated and proved.

1 - That (barring the writer's own work), there exists today no other fundamental system, no other standard code, designed to gauge, measure and indicate what really constitutes health normalcy. My method, in that respect, is unique and revolutionary. It stands out all by itself.

2 - That not even the medical fraternity as a profession really understand the natural laws of life as applied to normal living, hence the reason for that profession's failure to benefit civilization by proper teaching of health control.

3 - That there is today probably not even a single resident professor, scientist or doctor who is really enjoying normal health.

4 - That there is today probably not a single private or hospital nurse, or private or professional masseur or masseuse, pseudo or bona-fide physical culture director, who can properly and fully explain what constitutes normal health, and who is a living example of that natural philosophy of health.

5 - That in view of the foregoing facts, it is humanly impossible for these uninformed authorities to appreciate the condition, appearance and reactions of the human body in normal health at any age.

6 - That the teachers of our children are, generally speaking, usually not enjoying ideal health and wholly unable to detect (and therefore unable to correct) the unnatural, harmful habits acquired by their pupils.

7 - That not even the very trainers of our athletes, as well as our outstanding athletes themselves, are with only few exceptions, in any more favorable condition than their fellow creatures, and these often are not even aware of the superior standards of their own condition, which was reached not because of, but in spite of, their lack of information relating to natural methods innocently practiced without their knowledge. They attained their condition rather through the medium of artificial exercises, etc., to which they resorted in striving to realize their ambition to reach the heights

8

of physical perfection, thus resulting in their acquiring more balance of mind and body, than is found in the average person.

8 - That practically all human ailments are directly traceable to wrong habits which can only be corrected through the immediate adoption of right (natural, normal) habits.

9 - That the present-day efforts of our so-called health departments are in vain so far as physical health is concerned.

10 - That this condition will prevail until such time as marks the recognition of a standard foundation of sound and sane physical culture, based upon the natural laws of life, as applied to the coordination of physical and mental activities tending to the intelligent development of normal health.

11 - That all tuberculosis and a veritable legion of other minor ills, not to mention bow-legs, knock-knees, flat feet and curvature of the spine, and heart disease can be prevented (an impossibility under present methods).

12 - That the millions of dollars today foolishly expended in the purchase and maintenance of gymnasium equipment, etc., could be more wisely expended for the purpose of training teachers, living examples of normal health, not mere preachers of what normal health (if they really knew) should be.

13 - That the millions of dollars today spent on so-called health foods, health talks, and health articles, are actually wasted for the reason that the claims made for them cannot be proved.

14 - That comparatively speaking, only a very small fraction of the money now so spent would, if spent in the right direction, accomplish that most desirable of all aims; namely, restoring the population to normal health, naturally.

15 - That century after century we persisted in sitting and sleeping in unscientifically constructed chairs and beds.

16 - That only today has science discovered that the real cause of our restlessness lies in the fact that our modern chairs, benches and beds are so designed that comfort and relaxation can be had only by constant change of position.

17 - That our chairs, benches, settees, sofas, couches and beds seemingly are designed for every other purpose than that of

rest, relaxation or sleep - they are in reality the primary cause of our acquiring wrong and harmful postural habits, too numerous for mention here.

18 - That as with chairs and beds, etc., our physical training and sports, with relation to health, are misunderstood.

19 - That only through the attainment of perfect balance of mind and body, can one appreciate what really constitutes normal health.

20 - That for over 25 years, the writer has conducted progressive experiments along scientific and practical lines with his own body and those of his pupils, and the complete results of his extensive research along these lines, are now incorporated in the writer's work under his coined name of "Contrology." This represents a brief but comprehensive system of physical culture and is presented in the form of a new art and science, which, if universally adopted and taught in all our educational institutions, will not only tend greatly to eliminate needless human suffering, but will also tend to reduce the necessity for more hospitals, more sanitariums, more homes for the crippled, more lunatic asylums, more reformatories and more prisons. It also will tend to make the expression "health" and "happiness" something more than mere words indicating theoretical conditions rather than the conditions in fact.

Everyone possessing the moral courage owes it to himself and to humanity to investigate the merits claimed for "Contrology" by me.

Chapter 2: Health — A Normal-Natural Condition

GENERALLY speaking, the less the average person merely *talks* about health, the better it is for his health. Not only is health a normal condition, but it is a duty not only to attain but to maintain it. If human beings only knew and only obeyed the simple laws of nature, universal health would follow and the Health Millennium would be here.

Those more or less altruistically engaged in searching for, and studying methods to lessen unnecessary human sufferings, are compelled daily to witness the majority of their fellow-men unknowingly committing grievous sins against Mother Nature. They do this as if their very lives actually depended upon the success of their very efforts, altogether unconscious, however, of the fact that they are really jeopardizing and ruining their future health.

Imagine the immediate good resulting to untold millions, were the energies that are now so wastefully and positively harmfully expended, directed instead into the natural path of least resistance - the road to normal health!

Imagine how many more useful and happy years would be immediately added to their lives!

Imagine how much more they would really enjoy life to its fullest extent!

How many of us, or rather how few of us, realize what Life really is? Unfortunately, this ecstasy of living, is reserved for and limited only to those comparatively fortunate few who enjoy normal health - your birthright!

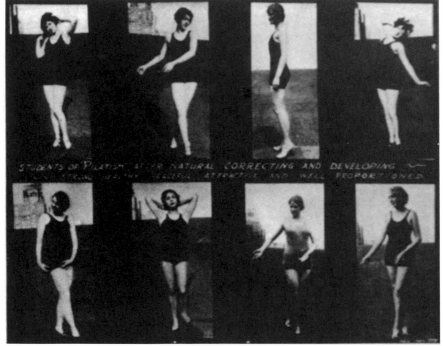

This is a most instructive chart. Here we see some of the girl students who had come to my studio at a time when they were sadly in need of body developing to continue their profession. Each of the persons on this page are professional singers, actors and dancers. I took them in hand and after three months of my corrective system of exercising, they showed the perfect form and posture seen above. Here we have concrete examples of the benefits derived from my method.

While recognizing that our modern system is to a greater or lesser degree responsible for present health ills, we shall not here attempt to indicate specifically wherein the fault lies. Suffice it to say, that the majority of our so-called intelligent men and women are so utterly and helplessly ignorant of the really simple laws of nature, that in their pitiful searching for normal health and happiness, one invariably finds them needlessly and heedlessly wandering about aimlessly and hopelessly. They meander through the valleys of quackery pointing ever downward to suffering, misery and death, instead of climbing to the very pinnacle of the mountain crests of common sense which lead to normal health, happiness and life.

Were the ailing "traveler" in life not lured by these mirages of false hopes, is it not logical to assume that he would ignore them entirely and courageously about-face and wend his way in the opposite direction? But who is there to warn him against these "mirages" and guide him to the "oasis" of normal health knowledge? These deplorable conditions cannot be attributed either to a want of understanding of natural laws, or their practical and beneficial application to the alleviation and cure of the ills of humanity - an understanding that really corrects causes rather than merely treats symptoms.

Never in history have more "time" and "money" been expended to attain normal physical perfection than in the present era! Never before have vain cravings for normal health been more justified than today!

Great military victories, moral triumphs, scientific achievements and industrial progress are indelibly engraved in the memory of men!

Business men, both during and after the war, were so busily engaged in piling up fortunes, that they entirely neglected to devote the necessary time to safeguard their health. Only too late did it finally dawn upon them that in the acquirement of their material fortunes, they, at the same time, carelessly and unthinkingly sacrificed the priceless jewel of their mental happiness, crowned with its physical setting of normal health, which they had so wantonly dissipated. Moreover, they also noted that their relatives and friends, who had followed "The Easiest Way" to fortune so-called, were continually complaining about the state of their poor health. They saw them pass the remainder of their shortened and spoiled lives, either in constant physical pain or in mental suffering, or both. In many cases they saw them die in the prime of life.

The mistreated body, mindful of its past neglect, eventually exacts its repayment in full with interest in the form of leaving business men their fortunes to contemplate, but denying them the benefits and enjoyments that accrue to other men of wealth blessed with normal health. The bitter lesson has been learned - but too late!

While business men now fully realize that "Everyone Is the Architect of His Own Happiness," they also learn that happiness is primarily dependent upon normal health and not per se upon the mere attainment of social position or monetary wealth. They have learned from practical experience.

Was it not natural to expect that under these inviting circumstances, so-called health specialists, common quacks, proprietors of patent medicines and manufacturers of various forms of mechanical apparatus - lamps, rollers, massaging belts, rowing machines, nostrums, serum and other injections, should, through their advertisements - lure the weaklings? Each quack assures the public that his is the ONLY method of quickly restoring one's health, and he bends his mercenary energies toward reaping the bountiful harvest awaiting him from the lure of the unfortunates, in the form of payments of unwarranted sums for treatments, remedies and services. Such treatments not only fail to accomplish the results desired, but in many cases actually do more harm than good, always, however, the good benefiting only the advertisers at the expense of his innocent victims.

What does this nonsense accomplish? It extracts money from the public without corresponding benefit to the public and for good measure, more often than not, adds to their suffering and misery.

It is very doubtful, indeed, whether a really sane and intelligent person would even think of attempting to prove that any of these many highly recommended "cures" accomplish one iota toward improving the health of anyone, much less effecting a cure.

Pardon this thought - But is it not idiotic, figuratively speaking, to permit one's self to be led around by one's nose by these wholly mercenary, unscrupulous and irresponsible exploiters, who, through their misleading advertisements, fake references and unconscionable methods, prey upon the blind credulity of the public? Think it over, you saps!

Hocus Pocus *is* hocus pocus by any other name!

Under ideal (true) conditions, not only the general public, but physicians as well, will enjoy normal life.

Looking into the future, it is thrilling to those enjoying normal health, in the interest of suffering humanity, to think of the time when through legislative enactment, it will be compulsory for those advocating cures, to demonstrate the efficiency of their methods as reflected in their own physical condition and health.

I stand ready for such test. My method has been proved satisfactory in every detail. My course can stand the acid test before the most critical experts.

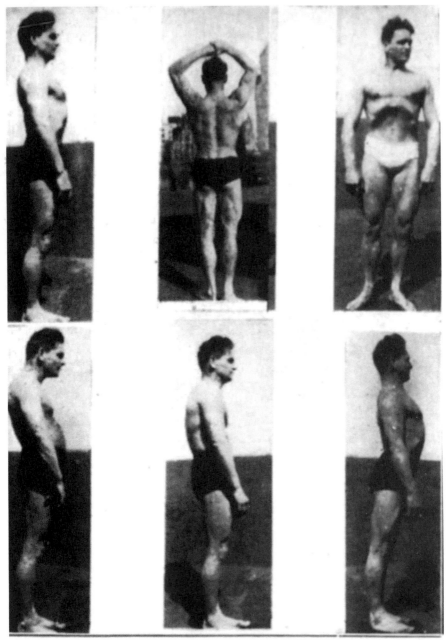

Here we see the correct and incorrect way to stand. Note the posture in each. On top we see three poses, front, side and back. Note the perfect body. Below we have the author posing first, in (A) the Macfadden Hollow Back incorrect posture; (B) the average incorrect posture of an athlete who is broad-shouldered and muscle-bound; (C) the usual position of ninety-five percent of persons, showing protruded stomach (and double curvature of the spine in both lumbar region and the neck.

16

Chapter 3: Dreadful Conditions

CONTRARY to the general opinion and popular belief that the mind is absolute master of the body, as expounded by Christian Scientists and others, and contrary to the general opinion and popular belief that the body is absolute master of the mind, as expounded by modern so-called expert physical culture directors and trainers who concentrate their efforts solely on developing the muscles of the body through the medium of various machines and other apparatus, it is contended that neither theory is the correct solution of our centuries-old health problems.

It is contended, however, that the correct solution of our present-day health ills can best be solved only by recognizing the fact that the normal development of the body and mind is possible, not by pitting the body against the mind, or vice versa, which results from concentrating only on the mind or only on the body, as herein indicated, but rather by recognizing the mental functions of the mind and the physical limitations of the body, so that complete coordination between the mind and the body may be achieved.

The theory advocated by this author is safe, sane and sound, whereas the other theories under consideration, are more or less unsafe and unsound. That is indicated by the newspapers daily recording the death of some of our most prominent men and women, comprising educators, scientists, inventors, physicians, industrialists, bankers, politicians, actors, lawyers and artists, who, more often than not, die in the very prime of their life. Unfortunately, only too frequently, when they are just reaching the heights of their vocations and when death overtakes them, deprives the world of their most valuable services.

Many of these notables silently suffer untold agonies for years, spurred ever onward by their own ambition to accomplish their aims, and while they themselves and their families are fully cognizant of their condition, the public as a rule, is in entire ignorance of it. These martyrs of false health doctrines die comparatively young, their families are bereaved, their friends are grieved and the world suffers unnecessarily an irreparable loss in their passing.

It is not generally known that many of our most popular misnamed expert physical culture directors and trainers, athletic and other champions, have suffered for years from all various ailments. Especially have they been subject to the dreaded heart disease. In fact, many of these persons die even before they have reached their prime, others right in their prime.

Barring accident, is not this record indicative of the fact that despite their expressed faith in their expounded theories and methods - and one must give them the benefit of the doubt - that they are mistaken in their teachings? Instead of improving their own health and lengthening their lives by the acceptance of practice of their theories and methods, they are, as a matter of fact, actually injuring their health and shortening their own lives, as substantiated by their own untimely death and the record of longevity established by other physical culture authorities, whose theories and methods are diametrically opposed to theirs. The system of the latter must be correct, since the acceptance of practice of their theories and methods by others, as well as themselves, results in improved health and resulting long life - oftentimes exceptionally long life. This is the "Nigger in the wood pile."

Very few of these exponents of physical culture can prove that their doctrines will cause one to live longer and happier than will one who never indulges in any artificial exercise of any kind.

Very few of these so-called physical culturists practice up to 60 or more years what they preach in their youth and very few of them can substantiate their claims as reflected in the condition of their own bodies whenever they do reach those years, if they live that long at all.

It would be exceedingly difficult to find them, for there are not many of them to be found. An impartial investigation would disclose that.

Now is the time for the promotion of a committee composed of influential personages, for the purpose of investigating the sad and deplorable state of ignorance existing with reference to one of the simplest, if not the simplest law of nature - balance of body and mind - and the absence of its practical application in our present-day program of physical education and training.

In these times, with ever-increasing mental training, the human system is more and more dependent on the vitality of the body, which vitality itself is dependent on the absolute coordination of the body and mind - perfect balance!

What is balance of body and mind?

It is the conscious control of all muscular movements of the body. It is the correct utilization and application of the leverage principles afforded by the bones comprising the skeletal framework of the body, a complete knowledge of the mechanism of the body, and a full understanding of the principles of equilibrium and gravity as applied to the movements of the body in motion, at rest and in sleep.

Lacking this knowledge, which is termed "Contrology", physical perfection, with resultant normal life, cannot be attained and comparatively early death cannot be avoided.

Unless the present-day system ignoring the art and science of Contrology are overthrown, it can safely be predicted that they will be successful in accomplishing more harm than good.

On the other hand, if the art and science of Contrology were
universally accepted and practiced, one could confidently predict that mental anguish and physical suffering would progressively decrease from generation to generation, and life would be a real pleasure, instead of the curse it now is to so many of our fellow men.

Therefore, it is recommended that the knowledge of the science and art of Contrology should be acquired by all.

Contrology is based upon lessons learned from a life-long study of the principles underlying and governing the laws of nature.

Suffice to say that incorrect habits are responsible for most of our ailments - if not all of them.

Equally true is the statement that only through proper education is it possible to correct bad habits for good ones, the time necessary, depending upon one's condition and age, and while the cost is comparatively nominal, one is assured of regained health arid renewed happiness.

Where can this information be obtained?

Who is qualified to furnish it?

He who criticizes anything without offering something constructive and proved, had better not criticize at all.

An idealist and humanist is in duty bound impelled constructively to criticize our present-day systems of physical education and training and prove by actual demonstration in his own body and that of his disciples and students, that they are positively harmful. He must lend his support to effect an immediate change, substituting the correct theory and practice for our current systems.

Accordingly, the undersigned offers - briefly to expound the general principles of his theories and methods covering balance of body and mind, upon which the science and art of Contrology is founded. He offers to demonstrate the truth of his statements to any person desirous of cooperating with him from a more or less altruistic and philanthropic view, in his aim to spread the doctrines of his system and furnish further detailed information regarding his personal ideas on the subject of "tension" and "relaxation," as related to the attainment and maintenance of normal health, so that the world at large may be benefited accordingly.

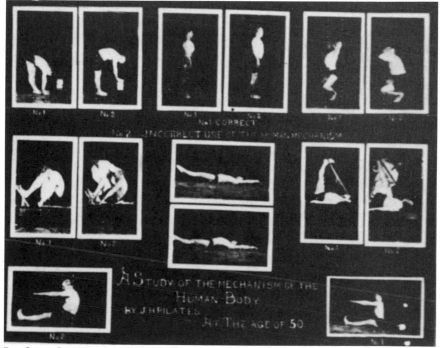

In this plate you see a student and the professor demonstrating the correct and incorrect use of the human mechanism. Study each photograph carefully and see how the body can benefit through my corrective exercises.

Chapter 4: Heading Downward

ARE we treading a downward path?

No, we are not "treading" the downward path - rather we are "racing" helter-skelter downward. We are slipping down a path that will lead to the ultimate destruction of the human race, so far as ever realizing the desirable goal of "Balance of Body and Mind" is concerned.

There is only one remedy. The public press must arouse interest to the end that such interest will compel science to "Stop, Look and Listen" at least long enough to permit of an impartial investigation of my claims regarding the simple, sane, safe and sound methods of attaining and maintaining normal health for all. Such an investigation would prove that my teachings will benefit humanity instead of permitting it to be exploited by the unscrupulous.

Science can at one and the same time eliminate poverty, ill health and unhappiness, if it will but investigate *all* and not confine itself only to matters close at hand and make bold to venture far beyond the horizon of its present narrow circle of orthodox activity. I appeal to the intelligent to put an end to the old system and to exploit my scientific system of acquiring and maintaining health.

As civilization advances, we should find the need for prisons, lunatic asylums and hospitals growing steadily less and less. But do we find this to be the case in this era? Certainly not! Teach the human race to care properly for itself and you will do away with these abominable institutions.

What a sad commentary upon our civilization to know that this deplorable "plague" can be annihilated if properly handled, and how criminal it is to think that the "cure" is offered but not accepted because of petty politics and jealousies!

Why boast of this age of science and invention that has produced so many marvelous wonders when, in the final analysis, we find that man has in the race for material progress and perfection, entirely overlooked the most complex and marvelous of all Creations - Man himself!

Were man to devote as much time and energy to himself as he has devoted to that which man has produced, what astounding and almost unbelievable progress would be made; a progress eclipsing all he has so far successfully accomplished, miraculous as that is! Just think that over, my friends.

Man should bear in mind and ponder over the Greek admonition - "Not Too Much, Not Too Little."

Man's neglect of himself, is destructive of his physical and mental efficiency and tends toward the gradual and progressive weakening of his morale with resulting ever-increasing dishonesty, immorality, loss of all true perspective of his responsibilities to himself and to his fellow man, with corresponding loss of idealism and ethical culture. Those are not mere words - they are facts.

Is civilization responsible for man's present-day physical and mental condition? This question is not so difficult to answer if we but try to see with the eyes of the Creator.

Granting that modern science and civilization do not materially benefit the savage from the standpoint of improving his mental capacity, still, at least, he is not harmed or "crippled" from the standpoint of his physical development. This fact can be quickly demonstrated by comparing the physical condition of an average "civilized" man with the physical condition of an average savage.

Logically, man should develop his physical condition simultaneously with the development of his mind - neither should be sacrificed at the expense of the other; otherwise "Balance of Body and Mind" is not attainable, and this very lack of harmony between man's physical and mental health, is primarily responsible for man's unfortunate physical and mental condition today.

If man persists in neglecting himself, or if man continues depending upon effecting cures with present orthodox methods, his case will be increasingly hopeless as time goes on.

Radically different research is necessary in order to discover and apply the laws of nature assuring man of his birthright to "Mental and Physical Balance."

"NOT MIND *OR* BODY BUT MIND *AND* BODY!"

Witness the splendid physique and brute strength of the average savage - his well-proportioned body is the very quintessence of physical beauty - however, brawn has attained the mastery.

Glance at the more or less deformed physique with corresponding lack of strength of the average civilized man. His malproportioned body is usually displeasing to the critical eye. However, in his case, the brain has attained the mastery.

What the savage lacks in mental development, the civilized man lacks in physical development. If their physical and mental deficiencies were interchanged without corresponding loss of any of the physical and mental assets each now possess, then the ideal physical condition and mental state would be possible of attainment - "Balance of Body and Mind" would be achieved. What a perfect specimen of human being such an interchange would create!

Relatively speaking, the savage is physically on a par with the beasts, while civilized man is below par, physically, but exceedingly above par, mentally.

Briefly, then, all we need do in traveling the "road of life" is to trace life itself from birth to youth and middle age to discover that which is responsible for disturbing and upsetting physical and mental equilibrium - "Balance of Body and Mind." Then it will be comparatively easy to recognize and understand the causes and to correct them according to the infallible laws of nature. In short, study your body - know its good and bad points - eliminate the bad and improve the good and what will be the result? A perfect man physically and mentally!

Before attempting to modify or reform any established practice or method, we must first know what is wrong before we can even suggest what might be right. Frankly, the indicated truth is that:

The average child is born of parents whose physical and mental balance was either deranged, or, perhaps, never even attained. Ofttimes, these parents are physically defective without themselves being aware of the fact, sometimes externally, sometimes internally, and sometimes both.

These physical and organic defects are not without effect upon their children, for they are usually inherited. A high percentage of children are born under unnatural conditions, many others, suffering excruciating pains in the throes of childbirth, and not infrequently sacrificing their lives as well.

Under such unfavorable birth, children are literally born to suffer, and much of the resultant unnecessary suffering is properly charged to the physical condition of the parents.

Enumerating a few of the more flagrant faults in man which brings on diseased children, malformation in arms or feet, weak bodies and other things are:

- Feeding children artificial substitutes for mother's milk.
- Feeding children when they are not hungry.
- Overdressing children when they are not cold.
- Forcing children to go to sleep when they are not sleepy.
- Stretching and bending children's arms and legs when they are not inclined to stretch or bend them.
- Compelling children to stand up when they are not strong enough to support their own weight.
- Forcing children to walk when they are not strong enough to control their physical movements.
- Compelling children to sit in chairs for rest (impossible so far as our present-day chairs are concerned), when they are not inclined to do so, preferring rather to "squat" on the floor Turkish-fashion.
- Forcing children to remain physically inactive when they are inclined to be physically active.
- Forbidding older children from climbing trees or jumping fences when their natural inclination is to do so
- Forced to remain quiet when they crave activity. Being compelled to study that which holds no interest for them and they make the pretense of studying simply to please their "blind" parents.
- Sometimes they are even taught to lie when their natural inclination is to tell the truth.

- Quite commonly, they are deliberately misinformed and taught things they do not understand.
- Children are vaccinated with "poison" to *keep their health.*
- They are forced to swallow laxatives instead of resorting to natural exercise to prevent constipation.
- Children are in these days of prurient prudery, either uninformed or deliberately misinformed regarding sex and permitted to gain such knowledge and information haphazardly in the street and elsewhere to their ultimate ruination in body and mind. Masturbation in both sexes, the curse of mankind, is the result of such handling of children.
- After completing their school day studies, they are compelled to study professions or accept such occupational employment as their parents decide in their "infallible wisdom" is best for them and except in rare cases of rebellion against parental authority, the "victims" resign themselves to their destined fate to the detriment of themselves and society.
- Children are impregnated with the thought that success is measured by the acquisition of money and therefore, their aim should be to become rich as quickly as possible.
- Children are in the same manner forced to go through the routine established for their physical culture education, which system of training is more or less mechanically followed without understanding and under the false impression that this routine is benefiting their health.

Millions upon millions live from the cradle to the grave without really knowing themselves and without really knowing what it is all about.

If they are familiar with the Greek adage, "know thyself", it is not practically applied to themselves.

These children in adolescent and adult life, lacking normal initiative, appetites, passions and the stress of competition, figuratively speaking, slowly sink to a low level, never experiencing the thrills of life, never experiencing the glory of successful accomplishment, and never enjoying the fruits of over-flowing vitality and health that should be theirs if taught the problems of life and the proper control of the body.

Later on, when their vitality is at low ebb, they begin to shrivel at their extremities, their blood pressure is either subnormal or abnormal - their heads get too warm, their feet and hands get too cold - their mentality waxes and wanes and they are, so to speak, more or less animated "clothes racks." This is a mighty serious problem. Think it over. It is deserving of every person's consideration.

And then again, they are influenced to join athletic teams, docilely submitting to a more or less brutalizing training regime, usually concentrating all their efforts on the physical development of the body and the acquirement of physical strength without any regard whatsoever to the acquisition and development of mental control. They are drilled to do stunts for which their bodies are unfit. While their bodies are either subnormally or abnormally developed, their mental control is absolutely neglected.

Is this the kind of instruction you want your children to have? Wouldn't the human race be better off if such system were abolished?

Do not all these violations of the simple laws of nature lead us to tread the downward path? I offer the human race in the place of the present orthodox methods, something revolutionary in character and results, "BALANCE OF BODY AND MIND" through the study and practice of the science of 'CONTROLOGY." MY SYSTEM DEVELQPS THE BODY AND MIND SIMULTANEOUSLY AND NORMALLY IN THE HOME, BEGINNING FROM INFANCY AND GRADUALLY AND PROGESSIVELY THROUGH SCHOOL AND COLLEGE DAYS TO MATURITY.

But will those behind the orthodox system of ruination, accept my new, revolutionary system of training? Not until public opinion forces them to do so, for they well realize that once my system is accepted generally, which must be the case soon, it will mean the end of the quacks, the crooks who wouldn't dare to undergo the very training they offer you as a build-up process to health.

Chapter 5: Common Sense Remedies for Common Human Ills!

WHETHER or not we are conscious of it, it is nevertheless a fact, that in the course of our daily activities, if we live a normal life, we receive the benefit of natural exercises - those performed in every movement we make. These very necessary functional activities, experienced by one living a normal life, preclude all necessity for undertaking artificial exercise of any kind.

It is really a rank falsity to believe that one cannot be both strong and healthy without having first to indulge in more or less violent training "stunts," but unfortunately this erroneous concept is so firmly entrenched in the minds of the general public, that it would probably require the omnipotent power of a deity to dispel this universally accepted nonsense from their minds.

However, in order that one may receive the maximum benefit and resulting normal health from one's daily activities, one should understand at least some of the more rudimentary underlying principles governing the mechanism of the human body in motion, rest and sleep. For example, the leverage possibilities of the bones composing its skeletal framework, the range and limitation of proper muscle tension and relaxation, the laws of equilibrium and gravity, and last but not least, how to inhale and exhale; i. e., how to breathe properly - normally. A knowledge of these are essential if we are to benefit from any exercises.

Since the public seemingly is either uninformed or misinformed with reference to these principles, they cannot of necessity benefit by them, which fact is only too self-evident when one, who is himself thoroughly versed in the knowledge of physical education, measures humanity in terms of normal health. If this knowledge were universally disseminated and the system advocated for its propagation, universally adopted both laymen and professionals, as well as by the properly constituted health authorities in particular, what a splendid human race we would see.

Again, the simple truth is repeated, that one may both attain and maintain perfect (normal) health without resorting to the expedient of artificially exercising the body. This statement seems to be fully substantiated when one observes the perfection of physical form, strength, grace, agility, endurance, health and longevity in the animal kingdom. With man it is just to the contrary.

Has the natural exercise instinctively indulged in by such "life" anything to do with the uniform attainment and maintenance of their ideal physical condition, as reflected in their natural beauty and normal health? Has the indulgence of artificial exercise advocated by man for man, anything to do with the uniform failure of his attainment to even reach much less maintain a similar degree of ideal physical condition, as is reflected in his natural beauty and normal health?

Would animal life benefit by exchanging instinct for man's ability to think? Or, would man benefit by exchanging ability to think for the animal's instinct?

Judging from an impartial study of their respective physical conditions, one must admit that were animals and men respectively to interchange their instinct and ability to think, that the animals would have bargained their birthright away for a "mess of pottage," while man would have gained immeasurably by the exchange, at least to the extent of physical perfection.

Did you ever hear of an animal gymnasium conducted by animals for animals, for the purpose of gratifying their desire or need for artificial exercising?

Is it not true that animals in their natural state and in their natural habitat exercise naturally as a matter of course?

Do animals understand natural laws and govern themselves accordingly?

The answer is "yes" because instinct unerringly guides all living creatures including man himself.

Have you ever closely and thoughtfully observed the movements of a newly-born babe? If you have studied animal life at all, you will have been impressed by the fact that so far as physical actions and movements are concerned, animals are men and men are animals. You see that in the movements of a new-born baby.

Both animals and men move their bodies in every and all possible directions - freedom of bodily action is paramount. This constant desire for change in movement in babies is only a manifestation of one of the many fundamental laws of nature - the law of action - which animals and human beings obey alike, if unhampered.

Natural instinct prompts mothers of the animal kingdom to permit nature to "take its course" as long as the lives of their offspring are not in danger. However, if one of the members of their sometimes rather large families seems to be inclined to laziness and disinclined to "play," its mother will not hesitate to force it to move about so that its muscles may be properly developed and strengthened through increased circulation of the blood. She will go even to the extent of grasping the "culprit" by its neck in her mouth and shaking and dropping it repeatedly on the ground until the lazy one responds to the hint. Have you ever watched a cat and her kittens or a dog and its litter?

How differently does the human mother act!

Instead of permitting infants and growing children the opportunity freely to obey their natural "instinct," as evidenced by their desire for action - constantly turning around, grasping for and holding on to objects within their reach, stretching and bending their little bodies, arms and legs; creeping on the floor and playing in the sand or on the grass until their little muscles tire naturally, and then fall into a healthy sleep as intended by another law of nature, the fond mothers literally stuff their offsprings' stomachs with food to overflowing capacity, and then "pack" their tender bodies in bandages after first (wholly unintentionally and solely through ignorance or misinformation on the subject) cruelly locking the joints of their hips and knees. In order to pacify their resulting crying protests against this rather inhuman treatment, the mother next proceeds to rock the child to sleep. Is it a natural sleep they thus get? No, the little innocents are either nauseated or half unconscious or both when they finally fall asleep from mere exhaustion.

How differently acts the dumb animal mother from the human mother!

The animal mother feeds her young ones as indicated by her instinct. Then she permits them to fall asleep, allowing them to assume their natural positions usually against her own warm body, which not only afford the little ones the necessary bodily resistance required for their complete comfort, but also gives them the benefit of the healthful magnetism of the mother's own body, an essential and vitally important factor in the welfare and well being of her offspring.

No college education is needed to understand what these remarks are meant to convey; namely, to observe what the "seeing" eyes see and to use common sense in the bringing up of our children. If only a very small fraction of the time and money now spent on research work were spent in the study of the many violations of the laws of nature for educational purposes, how much more would life be enjoyed and appreciated than it is possible to enjoy and appreciate life at the present time?

One understanding the subject-matter of this discussion may be pardoned for taking the liberty of discussing matters which are usually discussed only by scientists and doctors with degrees. Every free-born man endowed with common sense blessed with idealism, and prompted by humanitarian motives, instinctively feels it to be his duty to "cast his bread" (his own knowledge) "upon the waters" so that his brethren who may still believe in the observance of the ethical laws governing human intercourse, may benefit thereby.

Everyone is invited - no one is barred - to follow those in search of right and wrong and form his own opinion accordingly. In this instance, one begins his journey for knowledge, tracing it from boyhood to middle and old age, with the idea of testing the truth of these statements.

The child we left innocently sleeping in its cradle is now wide awake and lying on its little back, but, believe it or not, without the barbarous bandages, and with its hunger already satisfactorily appeased, it is enjoying the liberty of complete freedom in legs, arms and body improvements.

Isn't it strange that now, for some reason or other, we feel the same child unhampered by the bandages previously applied to securely lock its hips and knees when it was first put to sleep?

Most people seem to think that bandaging the lock hips and knees of sleeping and resting children is absolutely necessary in order that the legs may grow straight. What folly!

One never heard of animals resorting to this or similar artificial means for stretching the legs of their growing young and neither do we find savages resorting to such devices. Furthermore, since barring accident, we find the average savage and the average animal in nature in normal physical condition, blessed with well-proportioned bodies, and bow-legs, knock-knees, and double curvature of the spine conspicuous by their absence, we must reach the logical conclusion that the deformities children ordinarily suffer have been brought on by the terrible treatment they received as a baby.

If the reader has the ambition and patience to follow this discussion to its eventual conclusion, he might ultimately be convinced that adherence to this time-worn tradition of bandaging the child's body is really one of the first of the many bad habits which ignorant parents force upon their helpless children, a condition for which the health authorities are responsible.

The average normal unhampered child in attempting to gratify its perfectly natural desire for muscular movement, will naturally assume the so-called "spread-eagle" position, constantly stretching and bending its arms and legs, lifting its head up and down, and turning from left to right and vice versa. If left undisturbed, it manifests supreme contentment and keen joy, but after a more or less prolonged period of this state, it will begin to manifest evidence of uneasiness and unhappiness which condition if unrelieved, will bring on a crying spell. Then, if the cries are unheeded. the child will become exhausted, unless the parents intercede and change it to another position which the child is not strong enough to assume by itself.

Practically nine out of every ten mothers will confidently tell you that the reason the child cried was because it wanted to be carried in the arms, and this explanation seemingly is partly true, at least, because the child immediately ceases crying when its tiny legs are resting against its mother's body.

However, that is but another popular fallacy that needs to be exploded.

Why does the child really cry?

The correct answer to this question is quickly and definitely ascertainable. All that is necessary is for the experimenter to lie on his back in the same position as that assumed by the child and make the same movements for a period ranging from only 20 to 40 minutes, whereupon he will know what happens and then he will know why the child is restless and cries.

As it is, no one really seems to know what happens, otherwise this cruelty would have been abandoned long ago.

However, if the child were lying in a normal bed - one designed in conformance with the fundamental principles underlying and governing the anatomical balance of its bony structure - it could lie for hours at a time in any given position without experiencing any undue strain. Lacking the advantage inherent in such a scientifically designed and constructed bed, its position must, of necessity, from time to time, be changed, first from one position, then to another, so that if the child is found crying while resting on its back, the crying will immediately cease if it is turned to rest on its stomach and vice versa.

This change of position is now absolutely necessary for the child's comfort and if these changes be made at more or less frequent intervals, they will materially assist the child in the performance of its natural exercise, so essential and vitally important to its proper development. This procedure makes for the child's contentment and happiness and permits it to grow up strong and healthy.

Another form of mistreatment of young children is that of forcing them to sit quietly in a chair in a right angle (upright) position. What it really means to sit quietly in our modern dining room, kitchen and other chairs, for even only a comparatively short period of time, is something that those conducting our research laboratories have evidently failed to personally ascertain, for if they had, they certainly would have relegated the present type of chairs to limbo centuries ago and advocated the construction of the chairs which I have invented and recommend.

I challenge any person to sit quietly, free from all movements, for one hour in any modern chair. You'll soon learn what it means to the child. The muscles have become so cramped and numbed, that they are no longer sensitive to feeling. No one could really rest in such a position, because the position itself is a most unnatural one. For the naturally correct position, assuring the maximum amount of rest and comfort, it is suggested that one look around and watch the position that children naturally assume when they are left alone.

Does one naturally assume uncomfortable positions? Assuredly not. Then why not permit the child to "squat" on the floor, Turkish-fashion, American-Indian, Japanese and savage fashion, which position is at one and the same time natural, comfortable and healthful.

Children at this young age prefer and enjoy sitting on the floor, moving around bear-fashion on "all-fours" or creeping on their hands and knees, all of which develop the larger muscles of their backs, legs, stomach and shoulders.

Proud (and unintentionally cruel) parents, seriously interfere with and disrupt this natural course of bodily development by forcing the children to start walking or standing upright before their muscles have been sufficiently developed properly to support their weight and before they have the mental capacity to control their equilibrium in movement. Normal children require no parental instruction or help in this direction, for the simple reason that if they are left to themselves, they will naturally keep on learning and trying until they are able, not only to stand in an upright position without falling, but also until they have acquired the ability to walk by themselves.

To force children to follow any other procedure than this natural one, no matter how well-intentioned, is detrimental to the best interests of their health. Curvature of the spine, bow-legs, knock-knees, faulty posture and later on flat feet, are directly traceable to these mistaken ideas. They have their origin in the deplorable ignorance of their fond but ignorant parents.

How much more common sense or natural instinct have dumb animals?

34

How entirely different is their method of "bringing up" their young ones?

How much fun can we have simply by watching the animal mother especially of the cat family, giving a lesson in physical culture to her offspring?

What a lesson she can teach us!

Chapter 6: "Contrology"

The ancient Greeks probably knew better than anyone else, the true meaning of "Balance of Body and Mind," as tangibly expressed in terms of supreme physical health, supreme mental happiness and supreme achievements along the highway of human progress. They even believed that the soul itself is inextricably bound up with the physical functions and mental manifestations of the human body.

They fully understood that the nearer one's physique approached the state of physical perfection, the nearer one's mind approached the state of mental perfection.

They knew that the simultaneous and co-equal development of one's ability voluntarily to control one's body and mind was a paramount law of nature and that the unequal (abnormal or subnormal) development of either the body or the mind, or the neglect of either or both, would result in the complete failure to realize the very first law of civilization - (preservation of life) - the attainment and maintenance of one's bodily and mental perfection. Failing realization of this desirable aim, the body would become, as it were, an "'enemy" of the mind and vice versa, whereas the mind should become as it were, a "friend" of the body and vice versa.

Unlike so many of our fellowmen of today, the Greeks religiously practiced what they preached, as witness the marvelous state of their achieved physical perfection as reflected in their wonderful statues.

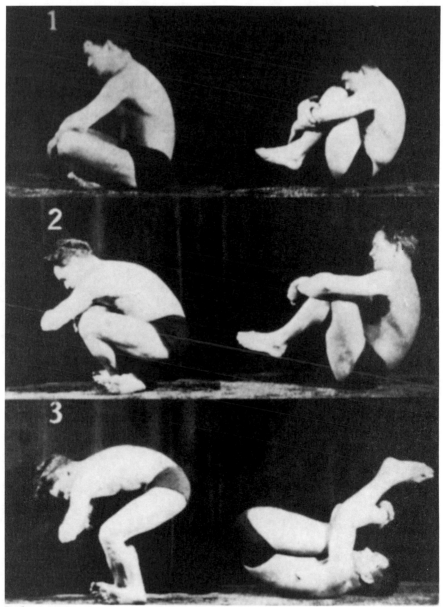

Did you ever try to get down on the floor from a straight to a sitting position? Try it. Having trouble? Of course you are, because there is a lack of coordination. Note the pictures on this page showing through Contrology the grace with which this can be done. Note the perfect curve, elasticity, and flexibility of the spine - the perfect mechanism of hip, knee and ankle joints.

In view of their unique physical and mental development, is it not logical that they should have established themselves as outstanding intellectuals and have been numbered among the "spokes" if they did not really constitute the very "hub" of the "wheel" of civilization?

Unfortunately for us all, their striking lesson seems to have been absolutely lost to modern civilization. What a pity!

With all our progress in many other directions, we still, so far as the harmonious and scientific development of our bodies and minds is concerned, have actually retrograded from their high standards of co-equal development of body and mind. Comparatively speaking, we are today really living in the "jungles of ill health and unhappiness", whereas the ancient days, man was living on the very "mountain tops of actual health and happiness".

The athletic prowess of the Greeks was continually being publicly demonstrated in their splendid and commodious athletic arenas, so that the masses could note the perfect bodies and seek to emulate the athletes.

Their beautifully developed and well-proportioned bodies proved an inspiration to sculptors, who immediately recognized the "living art" before their very eyes and perpetuated it in the unsurpassed marble classical Grecian statues now exhibited in our various world-renowned museums. That is one of the richest of legacies left to us by ancient Grecian civilization.

Truly are they an object lesson to us moderns that we should not overlook. Particularly should our duly constituted health authorities give heed to this lesson in health culture through recognition and practice of the fundamental principles governing "Balance of Body and Mind" in the attainment and maintenance of physical and mental perfection as the Greeks did.

The mode of living prevalent amongst the ancient Greeks was, of course, entirely different from that of today. These people were nature-lovers. They preferred to commune with the very elements of nature itself - the woods, the streams, the rivers, the winds and the sea. All these were natural music, poems and dramas to these Greeks who were so fond of outdoor life.

Their bodies were not unnecessarily burdened with clothing, as we understand it today. They preferred to more or less expose their bodies to the invigorating air and revitalizing rays of the sun, all of which, of course, made it possible for them to achieve their goal of physical and mental perfection to a greater degree than is possible today.

Were our athletes today to pursue the system advocated and practiced by these ancient Greeks, it is confidently predicted that with our present knowledge of "Contrology," they would not only reach the same high standard of physical and mental perfection achieved by the Grecians in their day, but as a matter of fact (incredible as it may seem), would actually surpass it, particularly when we view human nature "en masse" and compare it with the "en masse" standards established in ancient Greece.

The Greeks did not as fully understand the laws governing "Balance of Body and Mind" as it is understood by us today. Were we to discontinue much of our present mode of living and discard our present systems of physical training, and instead, adopt such training as I here advocate, based upon the science of "Contrology," there would result a rejuvenation of mind and body and living itself would again become an art as it was in the days of the ancient Grecians.

Habits of nature, rather than artificial training and exercises, would maintain one in perfect physical and mental condition.

Immediately following, I will explain in brief the general principles underlying "Balance of Body and Mind" - a science to which I have devoted many years' study.

Chapter 7: "Balance of Body and Mind"

A sound mind "housed" in an unsound body (50% balance) is just about as desirable a physical condition as is the structural weakness of a house boasting a fine copper roof but built upon a foundation of shifting sand.

A sound body "housing" an unsound mind *(50%* balance) is just about as desirable a physical condition as is the structural weakness of a house boasting a solid rock foundation but possessing a roof of flimsy paper.

A sound mind "housed" in a sound body (100% balance) is desirable just as is a fine copper-roofed house built on a solid rock foundation.

An unsound mind "housed" in an unsound body (no balance) is undesirable just as is a flimsy-papered roof house built on a shifting sand foundation.

What do the foregoing statements with their accompanying figures indicate?

Obviously, they clearly indicate that neither the mind nor the body is supreme - that one cannot be subordinated to the other.

Both must be coordinated, in order not only to accomplish the maximum results with the minimum expenditure of mental and physical energy, but also to live as long as possible in normal health and enjoy the benefits of a useful and happy life.

Chapter 8: First Educate the Child!

IN childhood, habits are easily formed - good and bad. Why not then concentrate on the formation of only good habits and thus avoid the necessity later on in life of attempting to correct bad habits and substituting for them good habits - oftentimes impossible even when the physical exertion is accompanied by equally strenuous mental efforts.

Therefore, it is of paramount importance that the child be taught the major principles of "Balance of Body and Mind." In other words, the proper development of body and mind, through the new science of "Contrology," is what must he taught the child.

Generally speaking. physical culture methods employed in our schools today may appeal to the uninformed laymen, but to one who has a knowledge of the subject, as I have, they would be amusing were it not for the fact that they are deplorable in their efforts.

In classroom and gymnasium alike (invariably either overcrowded or inadequately ventilated or both), we see children exercising a few minutes daily as a matter of routine.

Few children understand the significance of these insignificant movements of their arms, legs and body, and only a very few exercise with vigor.

The great majority mechanically exercise without mental concentration - an utter waste of time and effort. Such exercising leads to false conceptions and conclusions in adult life highly detrimental to the ultimate welfare of the grown-up child.

Before any real benefit can be derived from physical exercises, one must first learn how to breathe properly - this all-important function requires individual instruction, not only by precept but by example.

It is wholly insufficient to tell the individual to inhale and to exhale. To learn to breathe properly is really more difficult an accomplishment than the average (uninformed) person realizes. Moreover, there are comparatively few teachers who understand the art of correct breathing and who are capable of instructing others in the art.

"Carriage of the Body" is freely preached, but what the correct carriage of the body is, is not understood.

One constantly hears the expressions "heads up" and "shoulders back." In the effort to throw the shoulders back, the individual hollows his back too much (bow-like) and forces his shoulder blades against his spine, and most harmful of all protrudes his stomach.

That the instructions themselves are unnatural and without benefit, is of secondary importance to the fact that they are dangerous to one's health, which is of primary importance.

What really is desired, is not the backward throw of the shoulders as previously indicated, but rather the simultaneous drawing in of the stomach and the throwing out of the chest.

The average child (uninformed) when standing, hands in pocket, abdomen protruding, shoulders stooped forward, legs too far back, joints locked and feet at the wrong angle, is not being benefited by this condition as all of these postures, of course, are not conducive to forming good habits but are responsible for bow-legs, knock-knees and later on, flat feet.

Were the child in the first instance, taught the difference between right and wrong, he would naturally avoid what is wrong and follow what is right. Particularly in the matter of breathing, is this early instruction of vital importance.

In their normal (natural) condition, children do not need the stimulus of artificial exercise. Unfortunately, however, children born to live under the influence of the artificialities, require a special course in mind training in order that they may consciously control their bodily movements until the good habits formed become subconscious routine acts.

The first lesson is that of correct breathing.

Children must be taught how to take long, deep breaths, sufficient to expand the upper chest to capacity. They must be properly instructed how to draw the abdomen in and out at the same time holding their breath for a short time. Then they should also learn how properly to fully deflate the lungs in exhaling.

To properly deflate the lungs is an art in itself and this final step in correct breathing is least understood. As a rule, it is seldom, if ever, properly taught unless the individual is privately coached by one who understands what it really is all about.

Correct breathing exercises under the dominance of mental control, would undoubtedly accomplish more toward the prevention of tuberculosis as well as accomplish more toward attaining and maintaining maximum health standards, than all other remedies combined.

The lungs cannot be completely deflated at first without considerable effort. With perseverance, however, the desired results can be accomplished and with increasing power, gradually and progressively develop the lungs to their maximum capacity. That will actually cause the chest to "balloon" and at the same time bring practically every other muscle of the entire system into play. Thus the child's posture will then be normal (natural).

With proper breathing and correct posture, the child has no need for artificial exercise. Walking, running, jumping, tumbling, climbing, wrestling, etc., are natural exercises calculated by Mother Nature to develop her children normally.

The law of natural exercise precludes the hobby idea altogether in the matter of exercise, unless one is really and seriously desirous of not seeking symmetrical development of one's body.

For instance, the left side of the body must not be developed while the right side of the body is wholly neglected.

The law of natural exercises recognizes "companion" or reciprocal movements in the normal development of the body.

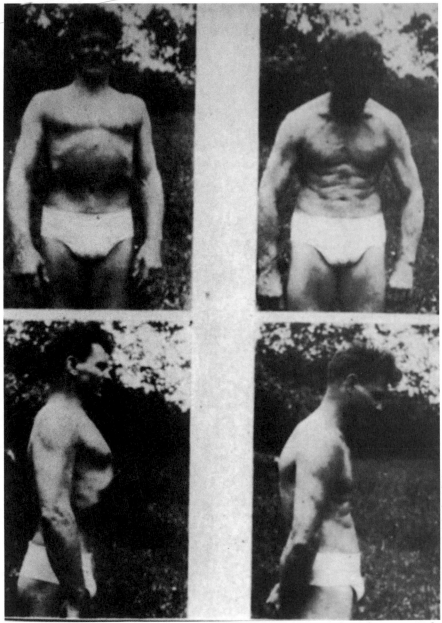

Here we have four photographs showing the correct way to breathe - two side poses and two front views of natural breathing. Note in each the chest at the point of inhaling and when exhaling. The first is the inhale movement, the second, the exhale movement.

For example, if a series of natural movements call for a definite number of forward bends, then this series should be repeated by a definite number of backward bends and so on, ad libitum.

"Hardening" of the body is another most important consideration in the matter of its proper and normal (natural) development.

Correct clothing plays a leading role in this regard. Children, if left to follow their own natural inclinations, without restraint, will not hesitate to discard unnecessary garments. In fact, the fewer the clothes, the better they like it.

The more active one is in outdoor physical recreation activities, the less need there is for unnecessary clothing. Children seldom, if ever, contract colds under such circumstances, but the moment these activities cease, nature prompts them to seek the necessary clothing protection to avoid chills.

Children should be permitted to exercise in the open air irrespective of normal weather conditions, barring storms and severely cold spells, because the open air is Nature's tonic that strengthens their bodies naturally and "hardens" them accordingly.

If the child comes home from play complaining of feeling a chill, or cold, it should be given a good hot and cold shower and, after a little rest, sent out again to rejoin its playmates so that its body may gradually and progressively become accustomed to its natural regime.

Many are the sins committed by uninformed persons in following false theories and methods for accomplishing this highly desirable result. The more natural and simple the method, the better.

Experience has taught us that it is the part of wisdom to practice very early in life exposing the young child's nude body to the air and sun as much as possible. No restrictions should be placed upon natural exercises so long as their indulgence does not indicate danger to health and life.

Much of the child's welfare depends upon cleanliness of the skin. Water should be freely used. Hot shower baths followed by gradually cooler and cooler temperature until the water is cold, has a most beneficial and exhilarating effect, especially when the body is briskly "massaged" (at the beginning) with a soft brush to be later on discarded for a harder one.

Soap should be used only occasionally as when the body is covered with perspiration. In all other instances, the brush massaging answers the purpose. This system of skin treatment not only is responsible for its soft texture and pink glow, but by removing all the soap residue lodged in the pores of the skin, opens these pores, thus permitting them to function naturally and eliminating the cause of colds.

Children should also be taught when washing or taking a tub or shower bath, to cup some water in the hollow of one hand and while holding one nostril closed, with the other hand, snuff this water up in the other free nostril, expel it by pressing both nostrils slightly, and repeat for the other nostril.

In this connection, if the water is permitted to enter the throat and ejected through the mouth, the throat and mouth are cleansed and kept in a healthy condition and gradually immunized against disease. These simple suggestions, if properly followed, would prevent the majority, if not all of our nose, mouth and ear ailments.

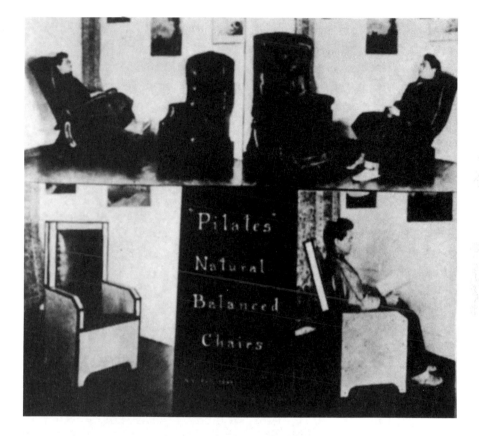

The above plate shows some of the many models developed by the author to insure correct posture and to rest the body perfectly. A chair for every purpose - from the kindergarten child to the aged adult suffering from the physical ailments so prevalent in old or middle age from the effects of bad posture and lack of exercises.

Chapter 9: Proved Facts!

PRACTICALLY everyone knows that nature has endowed human beings, and certain animals, with a "backbone," but few recognize that state of perfection which nature intends the human spine to reach through the medium of its scientific, progressive, and natural development from birth to maturity, so that the "ridge-pole" of the human "house" may properly grow into normal form (straight). Still less understand the mechanism of the spine and the proper methods of training this "foundation" bone of the body so that its movements will be under their absolute control at all times. Most persons are not aware of the fact that, by reason of this utter lack of understanding, the human spine has been sadly neglected, for many, many generations.

Accordingly, it has been permitted to develop itself, as it were, to fit the individual cases, with the result that the average human spine today invariably is more or less deformed. The prevalence of this condition, unfortunately, has been too generally accepted by the public as normal. Some of our leading anatomists, likewise, seemingly, hold similar beliefs. This state of affairs is truly deplorable since it not only gives credence to a grievous error, which, if not immediately corrected, will continue effectually to bar the victims of this gross misunderstanding from traveling the road to ultimate recovery, and prevent them from reaching their goal - normal health.

At no time in the history of medicine was it more important than it is right now, that organized science undertake an impartial investigation of the facts herein presented and supplement them by an intensive study of this all-important subject.

In view of the revolutionary inventions and the never-ceasing research in laboratory and afield, medical science should be emboldened to discard its old-fashioned ideas as well as its orthodox methods of instruction, and concentrate upon ways and means of preventing rather than curing disease. That is why I am preaching the sermon embodied in this booklet.

Consideration and examination of proved facts pertinent to

48

this subject should quickly convince unbiased medical and other authorities that the human body has for centuries been tortured unnecessarily by reason of our failure to recognize and understand the underlying principles governing the natural mechanism of the human spine, as well as recognizing and understanding the factor of equilibrium with reference to its application to the human body - in motion, at rest, and at sleep. That is a study I have made and upon that study I have invented chairs, mattresses and beds for the proper development of the spine.

It is the duty of the humanist to direct attention to this important matter, based upon observation and experience rather than to enter into merely controversial arguments with anatomists regarding divergent views on this subject.

Without undue reiteration (reference to standard medical literature is readily accessible) to the subject of these remarks - "the anatomy of the human spine" - the following is presented:

1 - Knowledge based upon fact regarding the mechanism of the human spine is woefully insufficient. This deplorable lack of knowledge is primarily responsible for the present-day acceptance of abnormal and subnormal conditions as normal, which in turn is responsible for practically every ailment afflicting mankind today.

2 - Spine curves as depicted by anatomists, represent on the average the actual conditions usually found in the human body, but instead of being accepted as normal, should be rightfully considered either abnormal or subnormal as the case may be.

Practically 95 per cent out of every one hundred persons examined are afflicted with an abnormal spine curvature. See photograph No. 1.

Undoubtedly, it is this very "preponderance of evidence," the 95 percent of malformation of spines, which leads anatomists and others to the false conclusion that since so many have this curvature, that represents the ideal and therefore the normal condition of the human spine.

Furthermore, it is contended that this curving of the spine is necessary not only to lend added strength to the spine itself, hut also that it may better absorb vibrations to which it is constantly subjected.

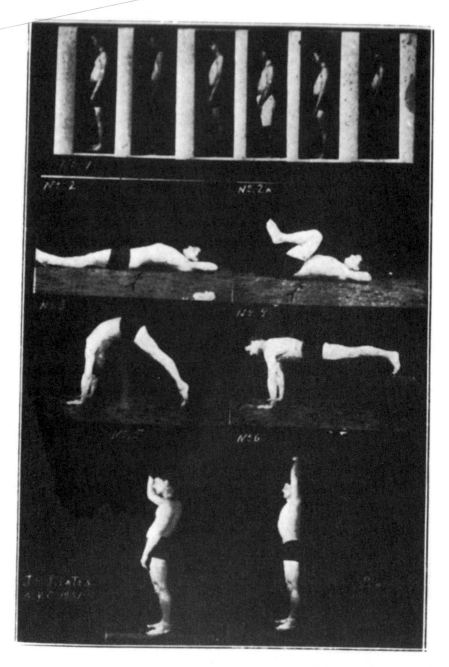

Photographs 1-6: Here is a chart giving proved facts regarding the curvature of the spine. It shows that the spine must be straight.

Has not science grievously erred in this instance in view of the fact that its unqualified acceptance of this conclusion is in violation of the simplest law of body mechanics?

3 - The spine of every normal child is straight. The back is perfectly flat.

Fortunately for its own benefit, the growing child inherits sonic natural movements such as that of bending the knees and assuming the natural curled position in sleep. Thus the child--animal (pardon the expression), subconsciously seeks the most comfortable natural position affording its bones just the right degree of resistance to achieve this desirable result.

It is almost criminal, to insist upon the child lying flat with legs outstretched and joints "locked" in a bed equipped with our more or less elastic modern bedsprings as most parents do.

Forcing the child to assume these unnatural positions incidentally reacts upon several groups of muscles, especially the major muscles, which is reflected in their tensed or semi-tensed condition, according to the extent of the child's deviation from the normal-natural positions.

Naturally, this unnatural posture, is both uncomfortable and more or less painful, as evidenced by crying until the vicious habit of wrong position is more or less permanently formed. Later on, the child perpetuates this harmful custom when parenthood blesses it with children and so on.

How much physical damage and suffering are due to this unpardonable mistake?

Photograph #2, admirably illustrates the bad effects caused by this practice of unduly taxing the muscles by the resultant steady straining pull unnecessarily inflicted upon them and which constant pull tends to draw the spine out of a straight line - its normal position. As the child grows older and reaches the walking stage, its spine assumes a more or less pronounced curve, particularly is this true if parents, through neglect or ignorance, permit the child to slouch, and deny it the benefit of natural exercise, such as creeping, and tumbling on the ground. These parental prohibitions detrimentally affect their offspring's normal development and jeopardizes their attaining normal health.

Not satisfied with this inhibition, the "head of the family" and his "better half" make matters even worse by insisting that the child stand on its legs before the muscles in the upper portion of his legs and the muscles of its back are sufficiently developed to support its weight.

These muscles are developed naturally and normally by permitting the child to run on "all fours" bear fashion, or at least by allowing it to creep on its hands and knees and after many trials with accompanying falls, to stand up leaning against the wall, chairs, beds, etc.

Every normal child, if left alone, will quite naturally and without parental help, try and try and try to move about from point to point as herein previously indicated. Knowingly to force the child to stand on its weak and undeveloped legs, is positively cruel.

The penalties are resultant curvature of the spine - are bow-legs, knock-knees and later on in life, so-called flat feet. The suggestion advanced that the curve in the spine affords additional strength to the vertebrae column, is scarcely borne out by even a cursory study of simple mechanical principles.

Photographs 3 and 4 furnish convincing proof that a lateral arch is undeniably stronger than a horizontal plane, while photographs 5 and 6 aptly demonstrate the fact that a curved line up right is **not** so strong as a straight line.

Therefore, is it not logical to conclude from the foregoing illustrations and observations, that there is no justification for accepting the curved spine as indicative of normal? Rather is it not conclusive evidence that just the contrary is the truth ?

Accordingly, by the same token, should not remedial steps be taken forthwith to correct the disadvantages arising from the continued acceptance of this false philosophy regarding the human spine?

The photographs submitted tell the story even better than the writer's words can do, since they are life examples and appeal to the eye as well as to the mind.

For instance, photograph 6 illustrates perfectly and furnishes adequate justification for the writer's conclusion that the normal spine should be straight to successfully function according to the laws of nature in general and the law of gravity, in particular. Photograph 5, aside from being unesthetic, illustrates only too tragically the ills inherent in the backward curve - decreasing force bordering close to no force whatsoever, mere feebleness, "dis-grace," the curve itself being especially dangerous to the vital organs and the body in general.

The slouch position illustrated in the foregoing paragraph (the pelvis is pressed forward), upsets the equilibrium of the body resulting in disarrangement of the various organs affected including the bones and muscles of the body as well as the nerves and blood vessels, not overlooking the glands. More or less permanently harmful injuries sustained, are not recorded here.

5 - Abdominal obesity and the dangerous effects of corpulency, have their origin in the "mis-carriage" of the spine.

Proper carriage of the spine is the only natural preventive against abdominal obesity, shortness of breath, asthma, high and low blood pressure and various forms of heart disease. It is safe to say that none of the ailments here enumerated can be cured until the curvatures of the spine have been corrected.

How can this cure be effected?

Unfortunately, the majority of those seeking the true answer, are still hopelessly groping in the dark after having read more or less false and true literature and listened to more or less false or true advice pertaining to this subject, or by reason of the fact that they could neither afford the time necessary nor the expense incidental to such methods advocated which might have proved beneficial to them. Only a comparatively few have learned the truth and benefited by it.

It is urged that the properly constituted authorities in our research laboratories and health departments impartially investigate the statements herein set forth, to the end that they may solve human ailments by methods of prevention and correction, rather than by methods of "cure." That is what my method of physical education does. I can convince you.

Time and progress are synonymous terms - nothing can stop them - the truth will prevail!

My work will be established and when it is, I will be the happiest man in God's Universe. My goal will have been reached.

Chapter 10: New Style Beds and Chairs

IT is scarcely believable in this day and age of revolutionary discoveries and inventions, that the constituted authorities of our Public Health Departments are so deplorably ignorant on the subject of scientifically constructed beds, couches and chairs of all types primarily designed to promote normal health.

That the correctness of the writer's theories in this regard is unqualifiedly supported by other reputable professional and lay investigators, it is only necessary to refer to the mass of pertinent information which he has accumulated during the course of his many years of activity devoted to the keen study and close research of general health problems. The conclusions reached by these various authorities as set forth in this booklet, are fully confirmed by my personal theoretical and practical investigations along these and similar lines.

This prevailing universal lack of understanding of natural laws of health, particularly by professional health authorities is astounding. In fact, it is unique in comparison with the remarkable progressive "Seven League Boot" strides of medical science, mechanization of industry, telephony, radio, television and so on infinitum ad libitum.

The vital statistics of our leading insurance companies indicate unmistakably that the death rate arising from heart disease is constantly increasing. Should not this alarming factor emphasize the urgent necessity for an immediate and intensive study of the underlying causes responsible for this most unfavorable and really unnecessary condition?

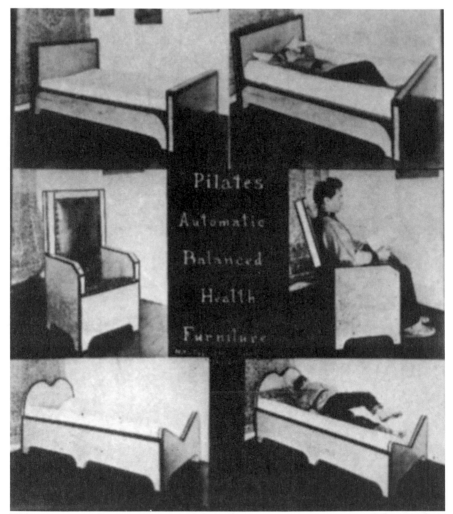

Here are a few more models of my corrective, restful comfort chairs and beds - each made by me in my studio. They can be made up in any kind of wood and any color to fit the color scheme of the most beautiful home.

While it is only too true that heart disease is not infrequently "acquired" in childhood, it is only too true that it is not often discovered until later on in life. Usually, the persons afflicted find it out when between forty to fifty-five years of age; unfortunately, often at a time too late to offer its victims a cure.

Today our public health and research programs do not sufficiently stress the importance due to a profound study of the "laws of mechanics" as applied to the human body. Particularly is this true with reference to a proper consideration and deep study of the necessity for recognition of the importance of the attainment of normal equilibrium of the body in motion, at rest or in sleep.

From a strict humanitarian rather from a purely commercial viewpoint, a close and unbiased study of the reasons responsible for the invariable restless tossings experienced by the average sleeper, can lead to but one definite conclusion with reference to our modern beds - i. e., that while admittedly they are appealing to the eye from an esthetic standpoint and apparently seemingly comfortable, they are, however, as a matter of fact, quite unnatural and impractical for the very purposes that they are supposed to have been originally designed. They do not afford maximum rest and complete relaxation. All they do is to afford a place upon which to toss the body.

Those beds may look pretty, but they absolutely fail in their aid to rest and health.

I have invented a bed that affords both rest and comfort, but the makers of our beautiful beds, will not give my inventions the recognition they deserve, for they fully realize that when this is done, the field of bed manufacturing will be revolutionized.

It is, of course, axiomatic that restful sleep is impossible without the fullest and complete relaxation of all our muscles.

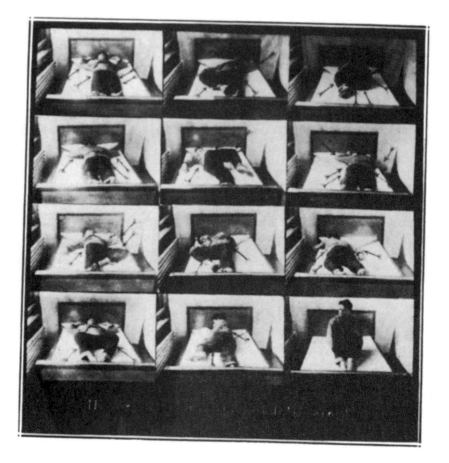

Here is the old style bed or the kind almost everyone is using today. The arrow shows the strained position in our present day straight beds. No matter how pretty a bed might be, it cannot and does not give you the comfort and rest of my "V" shape bed. There is nothing but continuous restlessness in the present day bed. All of the chairs and beds illustrated in this book, were made by myself, from carpentry to upholstery and each model is protected by patents registered with U.S. Patent Office.

Strange as it may seem, to those who are not technically informed, beds equipped with even the very finest of wire bed springs, actually defeat this very object.

Why? Because the bony structure forming the "foundation" of our body does not in beds so equipped receive the necessary natural resistance to afford the requisite simultaneous relaxation of both the skeletal and muscular systems of the human body.

Under these adverse circumstances, the body has, so to speak, literally to snatch rest with its corresponding motion of relaxation "on the fly," as it were. I have taken motion pictures of a person in sleep covering a period of eight hours, and my film, the same of that of the outstanding manufacturer of beds today, records as many as forty-five different changes of position during sleep. In fact, mine showed 48, and his, 45. In my bed, you won't change half a dozen times.

While recognizing the fact that we tire either by too little or by much activity - there is a happy medium - not too much and not too little. Is not an average of $5^5/_8$ movements an hour during sleep rather excessive for persons supposedly enjoying normal health.

Can the body under such conditions really receive the benefit naturally inherent in proper rest which is implied by minimum rather than maximum changes of position during normal sleep?

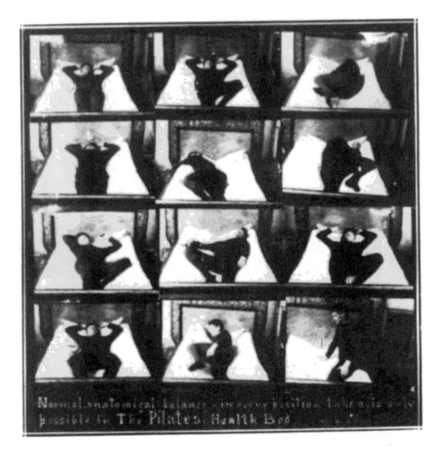

Normal anatomical balance in every position is possible in The Pilates Health Bed

Here is the author resting comfortably in one of the bed inventions. Note the manner in which he rests - like the cat or the dog in his natural, comfortable position. This is my "V" shape bed and has been specially devised for the child as a bed for correcting faulty posture and perfect relaxation of the spine and the muscles surrounding it. This "V" bed is especially adopted for the expectant mother, who requires all the comfort and rest she can get and also requires a perfect spine. This is the natural bed for the hospital for expectant mothers, asthma sufferers and consumptives.

Is it not perfectly reasonable and logical to deduce from this inference that our present-day beds are unfortunately neither designed nor constructed to afford the maximum of proper rest for the body? This deduction is demonstrably true. Here are the facts:

From time immemorable, it has been the stupid parents, wholly ignorant of the laws of nature, who have unknowingly inflicted needless cruelty upon their offspring. They have labored under the false impression that their growing children must stretch their little legs out straight while sleeping in their beds instead of permitting them to retain the natural and normal position in sleep. That normal position is one in which they entered the world. It is a position similar to that taken by the cat family and other animals when they curl themselves up in a "coil," just before going to sleep.

In this respect, it would seem that the instinct of the mothers of the animal kingdom is to that extent, at least, far superior to the unthinking practice of the mothers of mankind. Unfortunately, this is only one instance of the many "sins" against the laws of nature committed by the majority of mothers calculated to jeopardize the present health and future welfare of their progeny. Certainly if animals thrive on such coiling practice, mankind can do likewise. Try it and see for yourself. You won't suffer from constipation, weak kidneys and other ailments if you sleep as the cat sleeps.

Why haven't our educators the moral courage to advocate the immediate destruction of all the old and musty orthodox tomes which continue to perpetuate the teaching of false health doctrines? Why don't they actively advocate the immediate substitution therefor of modern physical culture books based upon sane, sound and safe methods such as I have preached in this book? Do you want the answer? Because such adoption would ruin them.

Why does practically every one naturally assume, what might be for want of a better term, called the "kitten coil" position when preparing to go to sleep?

Why do health authorities assert that to assume this natural position, is not only unnatural but also not conducive to good health?

What sound, logical arguments can be advanced to support the obvious falsity of the latter foregoing conclusion?

Is it correctly based upon any well known and equally well recognized principles governing the laws of nature?

Why is it that children and adults alike, whenever opportunity presents itself, invariably tend when seated to lean backward in a tilted position and balance themselves on the rear legs of a chair?

Why do mothers and fathers object to the foregoing practice (aside from the fact that doing so, scratches the chair and mars the wall etc.)?

Why do most of us become more or less restless and lean backward and forward, cross our legs from left to right and vice versa after we have been sitting in a chair for only a comparatively short period of time?

Why is it that it is more comfortable to "squat" on the floor, Turkish or American Indian fashion, than it is to sit comfortably for a longer or shorter time in an ordinary chair?

Why are present-day chairs and beds not what they should be - mediums for rest, relaxation and normal sleep?

The correct answers to the foregoing series of closely related questions are all of paramount importance and should be closely studied. You have them all in this booklet.

I will be most happy to demonstrate my system and my inventions to all interested. My aim is to offer a real service to humanity from an altruistic and philanthropic point of view.

I am not of the mercenary, quack type. I welcome the opportunity to furnish further detailed information regarding my personal views on the subject of "Tension" and "Relaxation" as related to the attainment and maintenance of normal health to all who read this.

I have the only course in the world that teaches physical education on a corrective basis and brings the results I claim for it. I have invented, as I already stated, several variety of chairs - one for the kindergarten children to build proper posture and keep the spine as God intended it to be; another for the benefit of those afflicted with knock-knees, bow-legs and flat feet, also a corrective chair; still another for the development of proper posture for the man who must sit at a desk and has little time for exercising; and a fourth as an aid for those who have been afflicted with the scourge of infantile paralysis and require leg and arm movements.

I have invented, as I have already stated, several types of beds and mattresses, which, those who have viewed them in my studios at 939 Eighth Avenue, have marveled at. Those beds and mattresses are so revolutionary, that when I showed a model to a leading bed and mattress manufacturer with the aim of having him produce them in quantities, his chief engineer remarked:

"Prof. Pilates, your invention is marvelous, but it cannot be adopted by us because if we did, it would mean turning our entire plant topsy-turvy. We would have to destroy all of our present-day models and create new advertising and that would practically mean starting out on a new business."

And immediately following that, this firm began to advertise extensively the very thing I had submitted - namely, that a person in sleep moves from forty to fifty times, and that by the use of their specially constructed mattress, such restlessness is reduced at least thirty percent. But do they? Certainly not! They still sell and use the old style mattress and bed. It was just a ruse to offset any advertising I might do.

What folly! I appeal in this booklet to those interested in the future welfare of our race.

I appeal to them to aid in putting my practical physical education method before the public where it will do most benefit, and to have them see and test my health producing inventions to the end that mankind can enjoy God's blessing - health and happiness.

Also Published by Presentation Dynamics LLC
The Original, Separately Bound Versions of:

Pilates' Return to Life Through Contrology
Original Version: ISBN13: 978-0-9614937-9-0

and Pilates' Return to Life through Contrology,
Revised Edition for the 21st Century
ISBN13: 978-1-928564-90-4
Available from Atlas Books (800-247-6553) or any book seller

Pilates' "Return to Life Through Contrology" represents the **first major publication in 1945 by Joseph H. Pilates and William J. Miller detailing the exercises, poses, and instructions** fundamental to the matwork developed by Joseph and Clara Pilates. Based on his concepts of a balanced Body and Mind, drawn from the approach espoused by the early Greeks, **these are the original exercises** that currently sustain a worldwide revolution in fitness strategies and exercise techniques.

Joseph Pilates has been nothing short of **revolutionary in his impact on the world of fitness and exercise**. You will learn in this book the original 34 exercises that he taught to his students, many of whom have become exercise gurus in their own right. These carefully designed exercises constitute the results of decades of scientific study, experimentation and research into the variety of physical ills that upset the **balance of body and mind**.

Pilates makes extraordinary claims about the benefits of his defined science of "**Contrology**". The exercises shown in this original book constitute the breadth of his ground-breaking definition of Contrology, and are basic to the growing army of worldwide trainers whose teachings rely on the instructions contained in this book. Living testimony to the validity of his own teachings, the photographs of this book are of Joseph Pilates himself at age sixty!

In this book, you will learn the exercises that Joseph Pilates recommended to accompany the basic advice found in his book, Your Health, regarding **posture, body mechanics, correct breathing, spinal flexibility, and physical education**. It is fascinating to study these exercises and to discover the origins of what is being taught by fitness enthusiasts, health educators, and exercise trainers around the world.